This is Not a Diet

by Graham Barrow

Table of Contents

One – Introduction 5
What I need from you and what you'll get from me 5
    Are you still with me? 6
    What can you expect from the following chapters? 7

Two – Weight 11
    What is your body made of? 11
    Your weight is not a data point 13
    Weigh every day 14
    In the beginning... 14
    My journey 15

Three – Metabolism 21
    Where does your energy come from? 21
    Basal Metabolic Rate 22
    Homeostasis 24
    Active calories 26

Four – The psychology of eating to lose weight 29
    Evolutionary psychology 29
    Distraction activities 30
    Finding the right pattern of eating 31
    Let's start doing some figures 32
    The easy to miss stuff 33
    And at the end of the day... 35

Five – Exercise 37
    Walking to fitness 38
    How fitness affects calories 39
    The acid test 42
    What about weekends? 43
    Other walking benefits 46

Six – Data 47
    My weight 48
    My BMR 49
    My resting heart rate 50
    My blood pressure 53
    Measurements 55

Seven – Bringing it all together 57
    The different elements 57

Table of Figures

Figure 1 - Male and Female body fat percentages 12
Figure 2 - My initial readings: the first 15 days 17
Figure 3 - My readings for July 2016 18
Figure 4 - My daily Basal Metabolic Rate (BMR) data 23
Figure 5 - My overall weight loss 28
Figure 6 - My first walk into the office 40
Figure 7 – One of my later walks 41
Figure 8 – Is there a tunnel under the Thames in Richmond? 44
Figure 10 – My first "Beets Blu" weigh in: 15 June 2016 48
Figure 11 – My latest "Beets Blu" weigh in: 31 January 2017 49
Figure 12 - My latest BMR data 50
Figure 13 - My initial heart rate (BPM) 51
Figure 14 – My latest heart rate (BPM) 52
Figure 15 – My blood pressure readings 54

One – Introduction

What I need from you and what you'll get from me

There are two things you need to understand before we go any further.

1. There is nothing revolutionary in this book
2. You need to bring four things with you on this journey. They are:
   - **Motivation** – and not just a little bit of "I'll give it a try" but a great big dollop of "This time I will succeed". We'll be testing how much you mean that as we go through the book together but be warned... if you haven't got that level of motivation, stop reading now. Put your Kindle down and go away. Because nothing in this book will work without it.
   - **Application** – you can't "cherry pick" the bits you like and ignore the bits you don't. There are lots of choices along the journey, but you need to stick with all of the element, not just some of them.
   - **Patience** – if you want to lose a lot of weight quickly, this is also not the book for you. When it comes to weight loss, "fast won't last" and will do you more harm than good in the long run.
   - **Sacrifice** – you cannot achieve anything in life without making sacrifices along the way. If you do something new, something in addition to what you are already

doing, you cannot create extra hours in the day to do it. If there is nothing in your life you are prepared to give up completely or do less of, then you won't find the time to do the things I'm going to suggest, and you clearly haven't got the motivation, application or patience to succeed.

Are you still with me?

Congratulations! You've just taken the first, most important step towards changing your life (or, at least, your weight) for the better.

I'd better tell you a bit more about me, too, I guess. After all, why would you trust anything I'm about to tell you without having a bit more background information? There's far too much stuff out there on the internet, in print and on the TV that simply doesn't hold up without me adding to the pile so...

12 months before writing this book I was 18st 4lb (116kg). Unhealthy, inactive, far too prone to eating the wrong amount of the wrong things at the wrong time. And, because I am tall (around 6' 5" - 1m 96cm) I got away with it (to a degree). But, as I sit here and type this, I am now 14st (89kg). That's a 4st 4lb (27kg) loss. I have lost six inches from my waist (40" to 34"), six inches from my chest (48" to 42"), my resting heart rate has fallen from the mid 60 beats per minute (bpm) to the mid to low 50bpm and my blood pressure is around 110/70. I'm 63 years old and I am now lighter than I have been at any time since I was in my late teens. That's a 45 year low! My risk of heart attack and stroke has fallen dramatically. I have way more energy than I've had for years. This change in lifestyle has worked for me and I'm certain it will work for you too.

There's something else you'll get from that last paragraph. I like data. This diet is based on data. Nothing too difficult or complicated or convoluted. I also have a predilection for utilising a polysyllabic vocabulary (I like using big words) but will do my best to rein that in. Occasionally there will be some words that don't have a suitable substitute (especially when we talk about your metabolism) but I'll try to keep things as simple as possible.

Along with data this approach is also based on science. Not difficult, hard to understand science but science nevertheless. And it needs to be if it's going to work. To be clear, I am not a scientist. Granted, I am an avid reader of science books (there are hundreds on my bookshelves at home) and, hopefully and rather late in life, I am about to graduate with a B.Sc. in Psychology from the Open University but that's it. Everything in this book has been learned through publicly available information and an enquiring mind.

Many chapters in this book include the science behind their contents and points you to the data that hopefully proves it. At every stage in the process, you can make sure I'm not just making this stuff up. I will include hyperlinks to websites that can verify the things I write about. As I said at the very beginning of this chapter, this is not revolutionary. But I do think that the people in life who succeed are the ones who really understand what it is they are trying to do and how to do it. And that is the goal of this book.

What can you expect from the following chapters?

First we need to talk about your weight. When you step on the scales what exactly are you weighing? That may seem a stupid question but it's actually really important. You do not have one single weight. It varies throughout the day, the week, the month for a whole variety of different reasons. Not everything inside you constitutes part of what I'm going to call your "core" weight. And if we don't get to grips, up front, with this part of our new lifestyle then nothing else will work.

After that, we're going to talk about your body metabolism. It sounds scary but it isn't really. Again, if you don't understand how your metabolism works, why you need calories, how different suppliers of energy (i.e. calories) work in different ways and how your body deals with them, you will not be able (with some help from me) to put together a new way of eating that will mean you lose weight and keep it off.

Then we're going to go into much more detail about eating patterns, diet, food types and the like. This is going to be interesting as there is no one diet type that works for everyone. One thing I am certain of though, if you are going to succeed, you have to enjoy this change of lifestyle because, once you've started it, there isn't a point at which it stops. This is going to be the new way of eating forever. There might be subtle changes as you go from weight loss to weight maintenance, but if you don't enjoy the journey, you will get off at the first opportunity.

Importantly, this journey does not involve special foods, expensive foods, hard to find foods or anything remotely similar. Which means that it should either have no impact on your current food bill or, potentially, save you money. If you're going to lose weight you will have to consume fewer calories and, for most people, that means eating less and it would be dishonest to try and think otherwise. The trick is to find a way to eat less and not mind. It WILL involve food you already like and don't want to give up eating, because at the heart of this approach is the belief that you won't stick to what you don't enjoy.

And on the subject of what you may not enjoy...

...we'll talk about exercise. This might get a bit tricky for some but hopefully, having already talked about metabolism and diet, you will see that the trade-off between these three things can work in your favour.

Then we'll have a look to see how technology can help you on your journey. This bit is not essential and you can still succeed providing you have some basic equipment. A decent set of scales and access to the internet are required. The rest isn't necessary but could prove beneficial (if you're that way inclined). I love technology and it has been central to my change of lifestyle but I know that others can and do manage just as well without it. The choice is yours.

Finally, we'll bring it all together in a closing chapter where you build the picture of your new life, with your new body and newfound energy. You can track the improvement in your health, your improving vital signs (if you want) and your diminishing inches.

Are you ready for this?

Two – Weight

If you ask someone how much they weigh they will almost certainly respond with a number. It might be pounds, stones and pounds or kilos (depending on where they live and how old they are). I'm rather old school British so I think in stones and pounds although I am rapidly learning to parallel think in kilos.

But have you ever asked yourself if describing your weight in terms of one specific number really makes sense? Suppose you go to the loo immediately after weighing yourself? If you return to the scales you will weigh less but have you lost any weight? Let's look at that question in a bit more detail.

What is your body made of?

More than half of the average human being is water. You've probably come across that statistic before but it's an important one. Men carry a higher percentage of water than women (on average men are 58% water, and woman are 48%). That's mainly because women have a much higher fat content than men and fat cells contain a lot less water than muscle cells. Look at the following graph and you'll see the average difference[1]:

---

[1] By US Government official site - CDC -
http://www.cdc.gov/mmwr/preview/mmwrhtml/mm5751a4.htm, Public Domain,
https://commons.wikimedia.org/w/index.php?curid=36767940

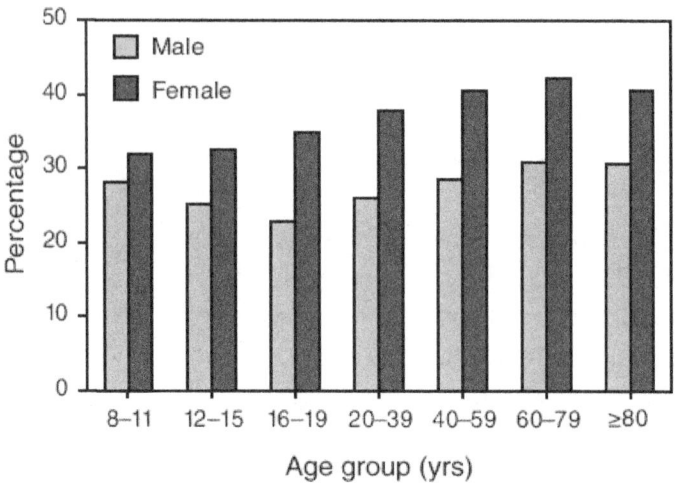

Figure 1 - Male and Female body fat percentages

After water, the rest of your body is composed of muscle, fat, bones, teeth, brain, nerves, body fluids and a few other bits and pieces intrinsic to maintaining your health. I'm going to refer to all these elements as your "core" weight.

But it also contains the contents of your digestive tract and urinary system (i.e. the solids and liquids you've consumed) and this is what I'm going to refer to as your "transient" weight as it can change considerably over a short period of time and doesn't, in my layman's view, constitute part of your "core" weight (although most, but not always all, of the calorific content are absorbed on the way through and that is where you can make a difference).

An important part of this journey will be to understand your own specific body rhythms (not to be confused with biorhythms which are something completely different). The passage of food through your body, the way we deal with fluids, how quickly they transit and how this varies over both the short, medium and long term will all have an impact on your weight loss and the maintenance of your new weight so it is important you understand them.

Let's go back for a minute to something I said just now. Fat cells contain much less water than protein (muscle) cells. Much less. About 10% compared to around 70-75%. Which means that fat cells contain much more energy (and therefore calories) because water has zero calories. We'll come back to this point later in the book.

I hope you will agree with me when I say that the point of this book is to help you lose "core" weight. It's easy to lose transient weight – just stop eating for a day or two and allow everything in your digestive and urinary system to empty out. The trouble is, as soon as you start eating you will put it all back on again – but neither the weight loss nor the weight gain have had any great impact on your core weight.

NOTE: To be precise, if you stopped eating long enough for your transient weight to have passed through you and out the other end, you would have lost some core weight through your basal metabolic rate (BMR – something we will discuss at length in the next chapter) but this is a bad way of losing core weight and will almost certainly involve burning the wrong type of cells in doing so. And it could also adversely affect your metabolic rate as well.

Your weight is not a data point

With this in mind, it is actually more sensible (although no one does it) to talk about your weight as being within a range, depending on where you are in your digestive process, the time of the month (if you are female) and much else besides. Lots of online resources will tell you that your weight can vary by a considerable amount each day, as much as 5lb (2kg) or more. Some of this is food in transit and some may be water retention (which can have a variety of causes – some hormonal and some through diet). I maintain a core weigh of between 13st 12lb (88kg) and 14st 4lb (just under 91 kg). I know that my weight last thing at night is about 2lb (1kg) higher than it will be the following morning (once I've been to the loo).

Weigh every day

Knowing your weight range and how it varies by the day, week, month is so important to this new lifestyle that the one thing which I believe is not negotiable is daily weighing. There is now a considerable body of evidence that suggests that daily weighing is fundamental to sustained weight loss but, to be fair, you will also find lots of people who say the opposite.

I can point you to a number of well documented reports that support my view, for example:

```
http://www.usatoday.com/story/life/2016/01/03/weight-
loss-scales-daily/77584478/
```

```
https://www.psychologytoday.com/blog/minding-the-
body/201312/daily-weighing-may-help-manage-your-weight
```

```
http://www.nhs.uk/news/2015/06June/Pages/Weighing-
yourself-everyday-helps-with-weight-loss.aspx
```

I will also relate my own experience with daily weighing (actually I usually weigh twice a day – morning and evening but that's just a personal preference).

In the beginning...

To begin with, you are likely to see significant weight reductions, particularly if your BMI is over 30 (More about BMI later). This is largely because early weight loss tends to be fluid based which can be fairly easy to lose. And seeing the scales going down fairly quickly is motivating.

As time goes on however, the loss will slow down and you are likely to reach plateaus along the way. I found that when my weight had gone up a bit on my morning weigh-in it reinforced my determination to keep to the new lifestyle. The thing about a daily weigh is that there is a limit to how much your weight can go up in 24 hours and it is always likely to seem manageable (and you can almost always link it back to either having eaten a bit more the previous day or, more likely – and there's no polite way of saying this – not emptied your bowels recently). I know that a full digestive system can more than compensate for weight loss over the short term but the trend will emerge over the medium to long term.

On the other hand, if you don't get on the scales for a week and, when you do, your weight has gone up, the demotivational effects can be devastating and it becomes much easier to give up and go back to your former lifestyle.

Daily weighing will also help you to understand your own bodily fluctuations. After a while you will be able to predict, with some accuracy, the fluctuations over time and they will become easier to deal with.

Let me take a bit of time out at this point to talk about my own weight loss journey.

My journey

On the 1st January 2016, I got on my scales at home (knowing I'd put on "a bit of weight") and was horrified to see an 18 at the start of the measurement. I had never in my life weighed over 18 stone and yet here, in front of me, was incontrovertible proof. I was 18st 4lb (116kg).

I decided there and then that I had to do something about it so I went on a "diet". And sure enough, over the next few weeks, I lost nearly a stone. Great! But then I ran out of steam and it all stalled there.

I was then hit, for completely different reasons, by a significant bout of depression and went into a bit of a tailspin. Fortunately, I had enough resilience left to do something about it and started walking as a way of occupying my mind and to stop thinking dark thoughts.

I started walking miles and realised that this was potentially a great way to reinvigorate my weight loss (which had stalled at around 17st 7lb – 111kg). But I also knew that the old ways of dieting weren't going to work so I needed to find something that would work for me. I'll tell you more about the diet element and the technology in detail in the coming chapters but I knew (because I am a data freak) that I needed data to make this work.

A bit of research threw up the fact that you could now buy Wi-Fi enabled scales which recorded, with reasonable accuracy, not just your weight but your BMI, muscle mass, fat percentage, hydration levels and bone percentage and would upload them direct to your smart phone. That was enough for me so I went out (or more accurately, logged in to Amazon) and bought a set. As we go through the book, I will post graphics from my own weight loss to demonstrate what I'm talking about.

Here is my weight loss from June 2016. The scales were delivered in the afternoon of 15th June and my first measurement, as you can see, was that evening. You can also see that the following morning, my weight was down by 1.7 pounds (allowing for a bit of rounding) which is largely attributable to my transient weight. However, over the next few days, you can clearly see that my weight was really going down. I didn't record every day's weigh in (although I never missed a day) as I only wanted to record the drops. I didn't mind seeing the weight go up a bit from one day to the next but I didn't need to keep a permanent record.

You'll also see that my BMI (which in January was over 30 – meaning I was obese) went from 28.3 to 27.7. Still overweight (under 25 is classified as within "normal" range) but still a useful reduction in the space of 15 days. You can also see my body fat reducing and muscle increasing – both good signs.

	weight	fat	muscle	BMI
evening 15 wednesday	17: 3.8	27.8	28.2	28.3
morning 16 thursday	17: 2.1 ▼0: 1.8	27.7 ▼0.1	28.3 ▲0.1	28.1 ▼0.2
morning 18 saturday	17: 1.4 ▼0: 0.7	27.6	28.3	28.0 ▼0.1
morning 19 sunday	17: 0.5 ▼0: 0.9	27.5 ▼0.1	28.4 ▲0.1	27.9 ▼0.1
evening 23 thursday	17: 0.1 ▼0: 0.4	27.1 ▼0.4	28.6 ▲0.2	27.8 ▼0.1
morning 27 monday	16: 13.0 ▼0: 1.1	27.2	28.6	27.7 ▼0.1
morning 30 thursday	16: 13.0	27.1 ▼0.1	28.6	27.7

Figure 2 - My initial readings: the first 15 days

I want to be quite clear at this point that I don't think that these scales are anything like as accurate as a set of professional body measurement scales are (like the Boditrax machines you find in many gyms these days) but that's not the point. I think they are reliable enough to show a trend even if the exact measurements are not necessarily correct. And the trends here are all in the right direction.

Nearly five pounds (over 2kg) in 15 days is great but I knew, realistically, that I couldn't keep that up forever. Nevertheless, seeing a 16 at the start of the weight measurement was a brilliant incentive to keep going. To be honest, at this point, I hadn't thought much past getting down to around 16st 7lb (105kg) and, all of a sudden, that target seemed to be in sight. In fact, it was coming into sight too easily so I revised my target down to just under 16st (anything that started with a 15!) although I was now toying with the idea of recording in kg and getting under 100kg (you see what I mean about the fascination with data).

Here are July's recordings (or most of them. They wouldn't all fit on one screen so I've lopped off the first few days – you can work them out from the previous screenshot).

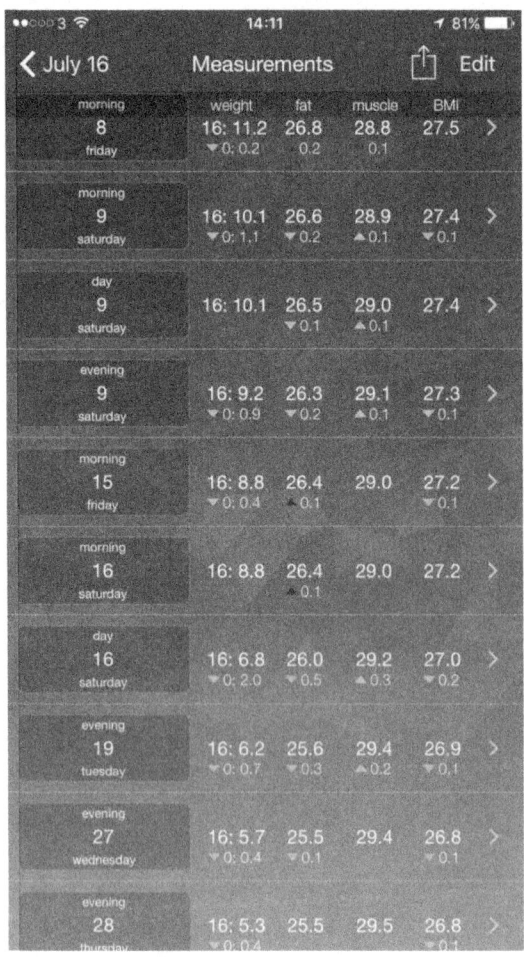

Figure 3 - My readings for July 2016

As you can see, by the end of the month I was 7.7lbs lighter than the end of June, having lost a further 1.6% of my body fat and increased my muscle by nearly 1%. My BMI had also dropped by nearly one point. There were occasional blips in fat and muscle percentages (but nothing to worry about) and the missing days were once again when the weight had either increased slightly or was the same. And, if you're wondering about the big drop on Saturday 16th, I went for a really long walk (around 16miles) and sweated it off – but it doesn't really count as, after I'd rehydrated, it took another three days to get back to that weight again. The point here is that on those days when it had gone up, I redoubled my determination to stick to the lifestyle I had chosen. Had I waited a week between weigh-ins, I am certain my application to the cause would have faltered and it would have gone up much more.

I'll share further screen shots as I go through the book. Partly because I'm proud of what I've achieved but also because I want to show you that this WORKS. If I can do it, so can you.

Three – Metabolism

I don't think it's possible to have a sustainable approach to weight loss, or even weight maintenance, without an understanding of your body's metabolism. So I'd better start off by explaining what I mean by metabolism and why it is so important.

Here are some dictionary definitions of "metabolism":

1. all the chemical processes in your body, especially those that cause food to be used for energy and growth[2]
2. the chemical changes in living cells by which energy is provided for vital processes and activities and new material is assimilated[3]
3. the sum of the physical and chemical processes in an organism by which its material substance is produced, maintained, and destroyed, and by which energy is made available[4]

Where does your energy come from?

You will see that the word "energy" figures prominently in each of these definitions and that energy is delivered to the body by the consumption of solids and liquids which contain calories (as opposed to, say, water, which has no calories and which is entirely

---

[2] http://dictionary.cambridge.org/dictionary/english/metabolism

[3] https://www.merriam-webster.com/dictionary/metabolism

[4] http://www.dictionary.com/browse/metabolism

useless at adding to the bodies energy store – but which is essential in order to keep the body functioning properly).

Importantly, around 70% of all the calories you consume are used in simply keeping you alive. By which I mean that all the vital processes going on inside your body; your heart beating, your lungs breathing, your digestive system working, your brain working, maintaining your body temperature; are all fuelled by the calories you consume.

Basal Metabolic Rate

And it wouldn't matter of you were to lie in bed all day and all night, your body would still burn these calories in order to keep you alive. This is called your "Basal Metabolic Rate" (BMR) and it's really important you work out what your own, personal BMR is. Fortunately, there are lots of online resources that will help you.

For example (my starting BMR is shown in brackets for comparison):

`http://www.diabetes.co.uk/bmr-calculator.html` **(2211)**

`http://www.bmi-calculator.net/bmr-calculator/`**(2210)**

`http://www.nscclinics.co.uk/slimming/weight-loss-tools/bmr-calculator/`**(2081)**

As you can see, there is a little variance between the calculators but they are close enough to work with.

This means that, if I do no exercise at all, I will burn around 2,200 calories a day. This compares favourably with the measurements from my Apple Watch (about which more later) which measures both active and resting calories. I'm not suggesting it does so with any great scientific accuracy but, like with all these data, it does provide both a guide and a trend line to follow. This my data from the beginning of June 2016. As you can see, the Apple Watch applies some sort of calculation as they vary day by day so I wouldn't place too much faith in them but, as you will see as we work through the book, as I lost weight my BMR decreased (which is exactly what you'd expect). I will update the figures as we go so you can see the impact that weight loss has on BMR.

‹ Resting Energy **All Recorded Data**	Ed
2,225	14 Jun 2016
2,369	13 Jun 2016
2,406	12 Jun 2016
2,447	11 Jun 2016
2,427	10 Jun 2016
2,391	9 Jun 2016
2,351	8 Jun 2016
2,339	7 Jun 2016
2,355	6 Jun 2016
2,474	5 Jun 2016
2,411	4 Jun 2016
2,387	3 Jun 2016
2,332	2 Jun 2016
2,398	1 Jun 2016

Figure 4 - My daily Basal Metabolic Rate (BMR) data

It is important that you understand this metabolic rate reduction as it means that, as you get lighter, you need fewer calories to maintain all your body processes and you will therefore either need to eat fewer calories or exercise a little bit more as your weight drops to maintain weight loss. It's not a big reduction but it's worth knowing about.

Homeostasis

On the other hand, and rather more encouragingly, now is the time to talk about homeostasis. I did say at the beginning of the book that there were some big words that were hard to avoid and this is one of them. There isn't really any other word that I can use instead so I'd better tell you a bit more about what it means and how it relates to your weight.

As before, here are some dictionary definitions:

1. the tendency of a system, especially the physiological system of higher animals, to maintain internal stability, owing to the coordinated response of its parts to any situation or stimulus that would tend to disturb its normal condition or function.[5]
2. the tendency of biological systems to maintain relatively constant conditions in the internal environment while continuously interacting with and adjusting to changes originating within or outside the system.[6]
3. a relatively stable state of equilibrium or a tendency toward such a state between the different but interdependent elements or groups of elements of an organism.[7]

---

[5] http://www.dictionary.com/browse/homeostasis

[6] http://medical-dictionary.thefreedictionary.com/homeostasis

[7] https://www.merriam-webster.com/dictionary/homeostasis

One example of homeostasis at work in humans is our body temperature. Normally it is around 37°C (98.6°F) and we only tend to notice a real change when our body goes through changes (e.g. illness) which are too extreme for our built in functions to control.

In the normal course of events, a part of the brain called the hypothalamus regulates body temperature through triggering changes to things like your sweat glands, and also the muscles controlling your body hair which can help the body get rid of excess heat, or retain it if your extremities are getting to cold. Actually, it is only your core temperature that needs to be maintained at 37°C, fingers, toes and the such like can, and often are, much colder.

So far so good. The interesting question is whether our weight is a homeostatic system as well. In an ideal world, increased calorie consumption would be matched by a corresponding increase in your metabolic rate so the additional calories don't cause you to gain weight. There is some evidence that this is true to a degree (for some people).

It is certainly true that you have much greater (but not limitless) latitude with your calorie intake when you are maintaining your weight than when you are trying to lose weight.

It is equally true that the western world has seen very significant increases in average adult weights over the past 20 or so years which means that homeostasis can only work within certain parameters and, for reasons we'll explore in the next chapter, modern human beings are finding it remarkably easy to overcome the body's natural tendency to regulate its own weight.

Active calories

On top of your BMR we now need to talk about "active" calories. These are the calories you burn, over and above what your body needs to maintain all your vital systems. And here you can exercise a choice. In a minute, we'll start talking about how many calories you need to consume each day in order to achieve a steady and sustainable weight loss and this figure can vary based on how many active calories you can commit to burning.

Let's go back to my own example.

As I said previously, at my starting weight of 116kg I had a BMR of 2,200 and I decided to commit to burning an additional 900 active calories a day. I'll explain how in a bit more detail when we get to the chapter on exercise but, for the time being, take my word for the fact that I had a plan that would allow me to do this.

That meant that I would be burning a total of 3,100 calories each day through a combination of BMR and activity.

Now I had to decide how many calories I was going to consume each day.

I decided on 2,200. That would give me a net deficit of around 900 calories a day or around 6,300 a week.

It is often quoted that each pound of fat you lose is equivalent to 3,500 calories so this ought to equate to a loss of about one and three quarter pounds or around three quarters of a kilogram a week. However, if you dig a bit deeper, you will soon find a number of articles on the internet that challenge the 3,500 calorie figure (and not in a positive way). And if you think about it, if it was true, you ought to be able to carry on losing weight consistently at the rate of one pound for each reduction of 3,500 calories consumed against calories burned.

But we've already seen that homeostasis applies to energy consumption so it is clear that the 3,500 calorie rule is just too simplistic. There's a very good article explaining the complexities of calorie reduction and weight loss at

http://www.todaysdietitian.com/newarchives/111114p36.shtml

The outcome of this is that weight loss is a long term endeavour that requires, motivation, application, patience and sacrifice. Have you heard that somewhere before?

What I can tell you is that I stuck pretty rigidly to my programme of saving 6,300 calories per week and in the 28 ½ weeks between 15th June and the 31st December I lost 45 pounds at the rate of 1 ½ pounds a week, although, as you can see from the graph below, the weight loss did not follow a straight line.

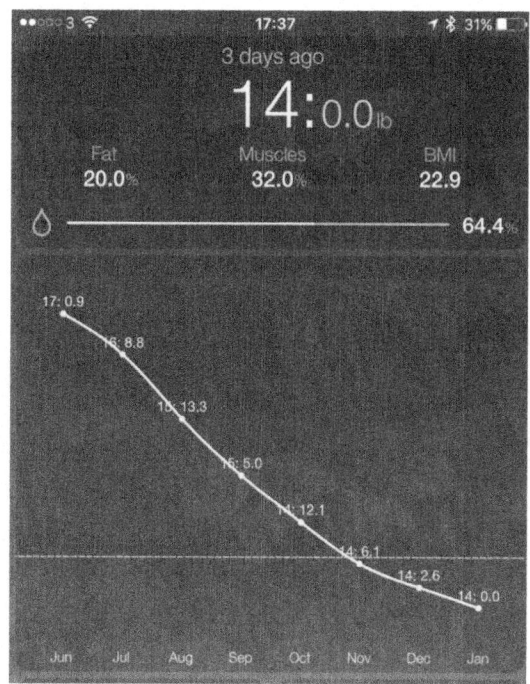

Figure 5 - My overall weight loss

Moving on, I said at the beginning of this chapter that metabolism is the process by which the body is provided with the energy it needs to allow you to breathe, move, keep your heart beating and maintain your body temperature (and much else besides). And what does your body need to generate that energy?

Food, of course. But not all food is metabolised in the same way, and some isn't metabolised at all, so our next chapter is all about how you can use your diet to help you to lose weight – and not just by eating less.

Four – The psychology of eating to lose weight

Over the last few years, with increasing concern about average weight and the explosion of diet books, being "on a diet" has come to mean something other than just being careful about what you eat.

Being "on a diet" creates an image of starting a special regime, consisting of specific (and sometimes quite weird) foods, for a defined period of time after which you stop and go back to whatever you were doing before (or something similar).

However, this book is all about creating a set of eating habits which you will use, in one form or another, for ever more. And if this is going to work, we also need to understand what the drivers are that cause "diets" to fail. So let's start at the beginning...

Evolutionary psychology

There's a lot been written about the Paleo diet, the 5:2 diet and much else besides, all based on the fact that our diet has changed much quicker than our genes can evolve to cope with. And this has almost certainly had some effect on our weight.

What is really hard to determine is "how much" and to what extent a change to a more ancient diet can help. And searching online will reveal a whole host of different opinions.

What is clear though, in my opinion, is that there has been a change in our eating habits, from a purely "life sustaining" diet comprised of whatever was edible and available at the time, to a social diet, where eating is not done purely for sustenance but as part of a more complex social interaction.

Which means that changing your diet requires you to address both the need to eat and the habit of eating. And they are not the same thing. Much of our day is now marked out by mealtimes – they have become the punctuation of our progress through the day with snacks as commas and meals as full stops.

The challenge we face when changing our eating routine is to be able to differentiate the need to eat through hunger with the need to eat through habit. And that can be very difficult. So I'm going to offer you a couple of ideas to help.

One is to think about what are called "distraction" activities.

Distraction activities

When you are trying to change a habit, it can be really hard to stop thinking about the thing you are trying not to do. One of the most effective ways of doing this is to plan "distractions" that take your mind off the thing you are trying to change.

This can actually be a wonderful opportunity to achieve one or more of those goals in life you have always promised yourself but never quite achieved. In my case it was to get fitter and so I chose to start walking. I'll tell you more about that in the chapter on exercise.

Finding the right pattern of eating

But, of course, you are still going to have to eat, and the challenge is to find an eating pattern that works for you. So I'm going to give you a couple of examples (mine and my wife's) which are quite different both in reality and psychologically but they have been equally effective.

Note: My wife joined me in changing her eating habits and has also lost nearly four stone in weight but, as you will see, although she has used the same structure, her choices within it were quite different.

I've always been a "lark" – up early and raring to go. My morning starts with a cup of coffee (I have an espresso machine which gets a great deal of use) but I also need to eat soon after my day begins. However, I need a breakfast that will then keep me going throughout the day so I have a high protein breakfast and I'll explain the reasons why in a little more detail.

Although, as a rough and ready guide, calories in minus calories burned equals weight gain (or loss) dependant on which is the greater, it isn't quite so straightforward as that. Different food types are digested at different rates and there are even some foods with calories that are not processed by the digestive system and go straight through you (e.g. fibre). In fact there has been some recent, quite surprising research done in this respect which I'll tell you more about in a little while.

Proteins are slower to be absorbed than carbohydrates which means they have the wonderful effect of keeping you feeling fuller, longer. That means that a protein rich breakfast takes longer to digest and helps you to get further through the day without needing much replenishment.

I am not a dietician, so I can't vouch for the overall nutritional value of what I'm about to tell you but all I can say is that it has worked for me.

I start most days with scrambled eggs, lean bacon and mushrooms. I love a cooked breakfast and never tire of having one and it keeps me feeling full right through the working day. I am lucky as my work often takes me to city based investment banks where they tend to have subsidised or non-profit making canteens where you can buy a decent cooked breakfast for under four pounds. But even if you are home, a couple of eggs scrambled, some baked beans and a slice of wholemeal toast is still a great start to the day and will likely cost you less than a large coffee from a high street retailer.

Let's start doing some figures

I'm a big chap (although not as big as I was) and, as I said earlier, I could allow myself 2,200 calories a day provided I also burned at least 900 through activity.

My breakfast calories were as follows:

3 eggs scrambled	275
2 rashers of grilled bacon	160
Portion of mushrooms grilled (250g)	55
Total	490
Balance for rest of the day	1710

My wife on the other hand didn't eat breakfast. I know there will be some who think this is a terrible thing but she found, from experience, that if she ate first thing it would, in her words "wake up her appetite". She simply found it easier to postpone the start of her eating day as long as possible as, that way, she avoided the worst of her hunger pangs.

She would tend to have her first food towards midday and she favoured peanut butter on toast. Her daily allowance was much lower than mine as she was lighter, had a lower BMR and, due to a torn meniscus in her knee, was unable to exercise as vigorously as I could. Her BMR at the start of her diet was around 1,450 and she burned a further 300 active calories a day giving her a total calorie burn of 1,750. She wanted to save 500 calories a day (3,500 per week) and so her daily calorie intake allowance was 1,250.

Peanut butter on toast is around 175 calories leaving her with 1,075 for the rest of the day.

The easy to miss stuff

At this point we need to factor on all those easy to miss calories that can make the difference between success and failure.

For example, I love my coffee and, although I always have fully skimmed milk I do have sugar in it. I used to have sweeteners but there is a growing body of evidence that some sweeteners may not be as helpful as you might think (for example: http://www.bbc.co.uk/programmes/articles/51yxBQyvqpNYPT3PF0LGL3G/are-artificial-sweeteners-bad-for-me) and anyway, I prefer the taste of sugar.

Each cup of coffee I drink has about 100 calories and I drink at least 5 a day so that's another 500 calories taken care of (you see how easy it is to lose count)! That leaves me with a balance of 1210.

My wife, on the other hand, drinks unsweetened tea with skimmed milk which is a whole lot less. Each cup of tea she drinks has about 25 calories and she probably has no more than four a day, making 100 calories in total and leaving her a balance of 975.

I like to eat fruit and I would do so through the day as a way of staving off my appetite until we had our evening meal. I guess I'd eat the equivalent of three apples during the day for a total of around 275 calories and a balance of 945.

And at the end of the day…

Fortunately, we both love salad (but not the boring old tomato, cucumber and lettuce salads we were both brought up on. A typical salad for us would look something like this:

Wild rocket	5
Celery	8
Baby plum tomatoes x 6	11
Beetroot	10
Sliced bell peppers	10
Chopped salad onions	15
Olives – green, pitted x 10	40
Home cooked ham – 2 slices	175
Boiled eggs x 2	160
Light salad dressing	100
Total	**534**

And finally, because we both really enjoy our wine at the end of the day:

2 decent glasses of prosecco	250
Grand total	**784**

So there you have it. A cooked breakfast, plenty of fruit and green stuff, wine to end the day and still within my target (provided I do my active calories).

And it worked!

If you go back to *Figure 5* you can see how I lost weight gradually over a period of 7 months, during which time I carried on eating foods I enjoyed, drinking my favourite coffee and wine but always thinking about how many active calories I was burning and how much energy (in the form of calories) I was consuming.

I mentioned at the start of this chapter that not all foods are digested in the same way and included the well-known example of fibre which, by and large, is resistant to digestion. There is another food type which is digestion resistant, which is called "resistant starch". Research has thrown up some interesting new facts about resistant starch. A recent, small scale trial conducted by the BBC programme "Trust me I'm a doctor" found that cooling and then reheating pasta significantly increased the quantity of resistant starch it contained. Which means that cooked pasta that is allowed to cool and then reheated prior to eating contains fewer calories than eating it straight from the saucepan. Who'd have thought? The full article can be read here:
http://www.bbc.co.uk/news/magazine-29629761

Now we've talked about what goes in, we need to talk about how to burn some of it off again.

Five – Exercise

Now I realise this is a thorny subject for many so I'm going to relate both my and my wife's experiences in relation to exercise as they are quite different and were driven by different requirements.

In my case, I was a fairly fit 63 year old when I started and was able to walk reasonable distances without too much effort. I do have dodgy knees however (from years of opening the bowling in local cricket teams) so running was not an option.

My wife had recently torn the anterior meniscus in her right knee (more commonly referred to as the cartilage) and, despite having had it repaired through keyhole surgery, still suffered some considerable discomfort so any great level of exercise was not really a possibility for her. However she was prepared to do a little bit as it was all going to help in the long run (or walk, as the case may be).

At this point, I'm going to take a small diversion and have a quick chat about Dave Brailsford. Some of you may have heard of hmi although many will not. Dave is the boss of the Sky cycling team and an advocate of the process of "marginal gains". In its entirety, it is actually the accumulation of small improvements which, when aggregated together can make for much bigger improvements.

I wanted to apply the idea, in a small way, to losing weight. It is the easiest thing in the world to think that one small cake won't make any difference, or not bothering to go for a walk when you really should won't really matter, but they do.

Let's say you have the equivalent of one additional, not really part of the diet, I'm not going to count this, well-known brand of individual apple pies, once a week. That equates to 210 calories x 52 weeks = an additional 10,920 calories a year.

And let's say you decide to skip one two mile walk each week which you have committed to and factored into your calorie calculations. That equates to another 200 calories a week or another 10,000 calories a year. That's nearly 21,000 calories which you have not burned off that you could have done. And that's probably more than four pounds (2kg) of weight you won't now have lost.

It's fine having the odd treat or missing the odd walk provided that you don't kid yourself that it isn't making any difference.

Personally, I used to treat these things like a balance sheet. For each debit I'd try and add a corresponding credit. Not slavishly, but at least try and compensate one for the other. If I went out for dinner with friends one evening, I'd try and do a longer walk the next day. It would be easy to become really fanatical about counting individual calories and it was something I never did but I would keep a rough tally to make sure I was in the right ball park.

Back to the job in hand...

Walking to fitness

When I started my change of routine I was working in the centre of London and I live in the suburbs. I needed to find a way of adding additional walking time to my day without seriously disrupting my working hours or it impinging on what personal life I had. And I needed to find a reliable way of keeping track of how far I'd walked.

One of the great things about the internet is that it gives you access to so much information at the touch of a few keys on a laptop or tablet. And, on top of that, there are a huge variety of wrist worn gadgets that can help you keep track of your steps, running time, heartbeat, and a whole host of other bits of data.

I started out using a Fitbit but graduated quite quickly to an Apple Watch (partly because I'm an unashamed Apple freak and partly because it just looked nicer). The great thing about the watch is that it collects and stores a wide variety of data which I can use to illustrate some of the things I'll be writing about.

In particular it tracks steps, distance walked, active calories, heart rate, number of active minutes and, as we've already seen, your BMR or "resting energy" as it appears in the Apple Health App.

All this means is that, one way or the other, you can work out how many active calories you are burning with a little bit of effort and an activity tracker or by using various website calorie calculators. For instance, there's a very comprehensive calculator at `https://nutritiondata.self.com/tools/calories-burned`.

I worked out that I could take the train from home to Waterloo and then walk into the City of London from there. My watch told me it was almost exactly two miles from station to office so if I did morning and evening that was four miles a day.

How fitness affects calories

Figure 6 shows one of my first walks with my new Apple Watch. At this point I weighed 17st 2lbs (109kgs). As you can see, the overall distance walked was 1.95 miles, which I did in 29 minutes 38 seconds (which is quite quick) burning 229 active calories with an average heart rate of 108bpm. These figures may not be totally accurate but they will be close enough to use as a decent yardstick. Now compare this to a later walk I did in December 2016 (which was slightly slower, mainly because there were more people around so I couldn't walk so fast).

I was now 14st 5lb (91kg) a loss of nearly three stone (18kg). You can see the effect this has had on the number of calories burned (and this is critically important). They've gone from 229 active to

180 and a total drop (including resting calories) of 57. This is nearly 20% fewer calories than I burned 6 months previously and is a great example of why weight loss plateaus.

As your weight goes down, it takes less effort to move around (which is good as you feel lighter and more energetic) so your active calories reduce. Your BMR also reduces, as your body needs less fuel to maintain itself. And this means that, if you maintain your calorie intake and expenditure, you will eventually stop losing weight. It might mean that, if you don't readjust, you start putting a little bit back on until you find your point of equilibrium.

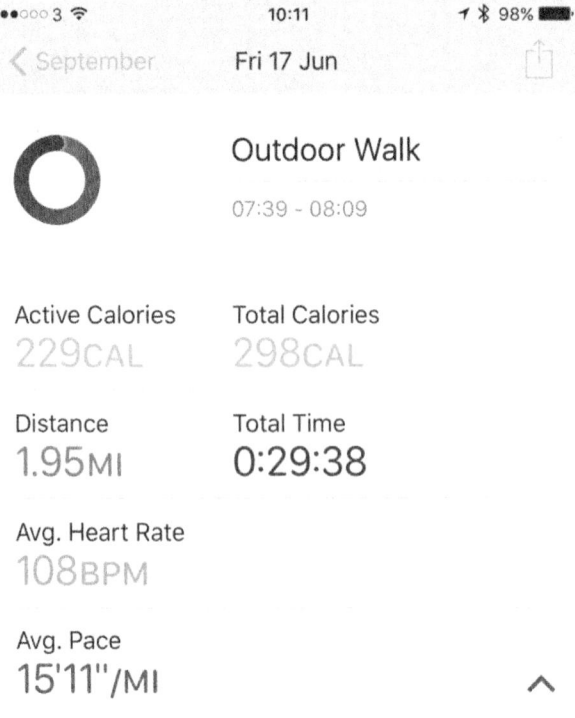

Figure 6 - My first walk into the office

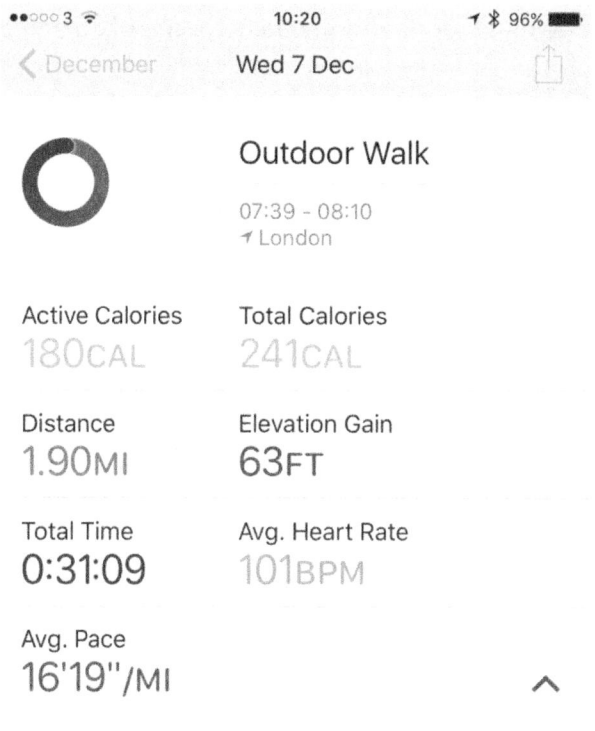

Figure 7 – One of my later walks

If you recall, I committed to burn 900 active calories a day and these two walks (to the office in the morning and back to the station in the evening) now accounted (at least initially) for around half of them (229 x 2 = 458 active calories).

On top of that, instead of eating lunch (as I'd had a full cooked breakfast already) I would walk around the city at lunchtime. On a good day I could do another 2 or 3 miles (depending on how busy the streets were) which would account for another 200 or so active calories (as an aside, a 180lb person burns roughly 100 calories per mile walked, fewer if you're lighter, more if you're heavier) Add in the walk to and from my local station each morning accounting for another 50 active calories and further 150 from the normal activities of being at work and my daily total looked something like this:

Walk to and from local station	50
Walk from Waterloo to office and back	450
Lunchtime walk	250
General daily activity	150
Total	**900**

My wife, who had far more difficulty walking, committed to 300 active calories which she could achieve, by and large, through her normal daily activities plus the occasional short walk. Interestingly, for someone who has never been that interested in technology, she also took to using a fitness tracker and now wouldn't be without it.

Even better, as her weight came down, her ability to walk became noticeably easier and the distances increased markedly. At the start of the year, it was all she could do to walk to the end of the road; by the end of the year, she walked with me to our in-laws for their New Year's Eve party (a distance of a mile and a half) and then home again (although that might have been aided by a glass or two of prosecco)!

The acid test

Do you remember at the start of this book, I said you needed to bring four things with you on this journey – MAPS:

- Motivation
- Application

- Patience
- Sacrifice

This is the bit where it really matters. Walking come rain or shine, getting out even on the days you don't really feel like it. Ignoring the call of the tube (fortunately, I hated the Waterloo and City line so this wasn't difficult) and keeping at it. These are the tests of your motivation, your application, your patience and your ability to make sacrifices.

Oddly, in my case, it made very little difference to the time I arrived at work or got home in the evening. I calculated that, by the time I had walked down to the Waterloo and City Line platform, waited for a train, got off the other end and queued to get through the ticket barrier, trudged up to the street level and walked in from Bank station, I only saved at most 10 minutes compared to walking direct from Waterloo. So not a big sacrifice.

What about weekends?

To begin with, when I walked the first few times in from Waterloo to work, I wondered how I was going to get the energy to walk back again in the evening, but I managed it. Actually, I found pretty quickly that things were getting easier and easier so I determined to see how far I could walk at the weekends. I am fortunate to live in a green and pleasant part of West London with access to Richmond Park, the River Thames, the Grand Union Canal, Syon Park, Osterley Park and many other lovely places – all on my doorstep. I know others are not so lucky but, nevertheless, one of the extraordinary things I discovered on my weekend walks was how many places there were locally which I didn't know existed.

There are some things that you only really see on foot. And allowing yourself the luxury of setting off without any particular destination in mind is fun. Go where the mood takes you and see where you end up. Sometimes they are dead ends but other times you find yourself coming home to tell your friends and family about some of the extraordinary places you've found right on your own doorstep.

One of mine is located on the River Thames by Twickenham Bridge and I still haven't really got to the bottom of it. Here's a picture I took:

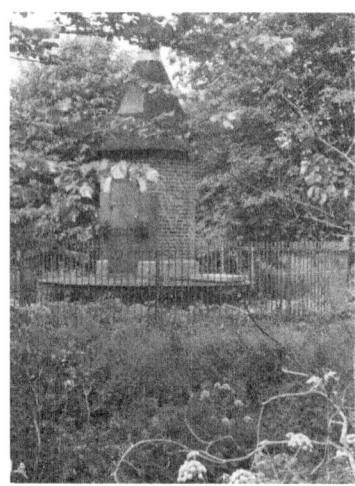

Figure 8 – Is there a tunnel under the Thames in Richmond?

There's an identical building on the opposite (Old Deer Park) side of the river. Research suggest that they might have been the entrance and exit to a long since closed pedestrian tunnel under the river but there's almost nothing available online to confirm or deny this. Which seems quite remarkable to me. And I'd never have noticed it if I hadn't walked.

My weekend perambulations became longer and more adventurous as you can see from this brief snapshot of my record of steps taken in late July and early August 2016 by which time I had, quite literally, got into my stride.

Steps	All Recorded Data	
32,026	6 Aug 2016	
14,412	5 Aug 2016	
13,669	4 Aug 2016	
12,817	3 Aug 2016	
12,358	2 Aug 2016	
17,975	1 Aug 2016	
22,666	31 Jul 2016	
26,246	30 Jul 2016	
21,600	29 Jul 2016	
18,319	28 Jul 2016	
13,768	27 Jul 2016	
13,370	26 Jul 2016	
14,616	25 Jul 2016	
18,703	24 Jul 2016	

Figure 9 – My steps for late July/early August 2016

The 6th August walk (32,026 steps) was quite a day as I did two complete circuits around the perimeter of Richmond Park (around 14 and a half miles in total) and was the point I knew for certain that my new fitness regime was working well.

Other walking benefits

There are lots of other benefits to walking regularly as well. In the next chapter I'm going to summarise the effects of losing weight and getting more exercise on my health vital signs but there's more to it than that.

I mentioned earlier in the book that I had a significant and serious bout of depression in early 2016 – one of those where you just cannot shake of the dark thoughts and the feelings of a complete lack of self-worth.

I know for certain that once I started walking every day, my mood changed, my depression lifted and I felt immeasurably more at ease with the world. Of course, I was losing weight and feeling fitter as well but I'm certain that the simple act of getting out into the fresh air (and occasional sunshine) made a huge difference to my emotional well-being. Studies have found that walking can change your mental state, reduce stress, boost endorphins and increase your energy levels.

As I write this, my data tells me that I have taken nearly six million steps since I started monitoring them, which brings me on to the next chapter – data!

Six – Data

I said at the start of this book that I love data. Let me explain in a bit more detail why and then let me tell you why I think you should too.

I have loved working with numbers for as long as I can remember. I know from my Psychology studies (mentioned in Chapter One) that I have, at the very least, Asperger traits and, more likely, I actually have a mild Asperger Syndrome. That's fine with me. I'm quite content with my lot in life and have no regrets at all.

Numbers have always seemed like friends to me, largely because they have a truth to them (as distinct from statistics which can be horribly manipulated). Provided my scales are accurate (and modern scales are pretty good) what it says on the display is what I am.

If I was born in October 1953 and it is now February 2017, I am definitely 63 years old. These things are without debate. Data tends to be neutral, honest and predictable – three things that can be far more troublesome when applied to human beings.

This chapter is going to be a record of my data over the duration of my weight loss period. My primary reason for including it is to show you that this process works, is beneficial and worth the effort. But, of course, there is a secondary reason – I'm proud of what I've achieve and this is a chance to show off and there's no point trying to dress it up any other way.

However, if I can achieve my primary goal of proving this works and satisfy my ego at the same time – so be it!

My weight

Let's start with weight, as the change in my weight is the most obvious outcome from this programme. Here's my first ever weigh-in on my brand new Beets Blu scales:

Figure 10 – My first "Beets Blu" weigh in: 15 June 2016

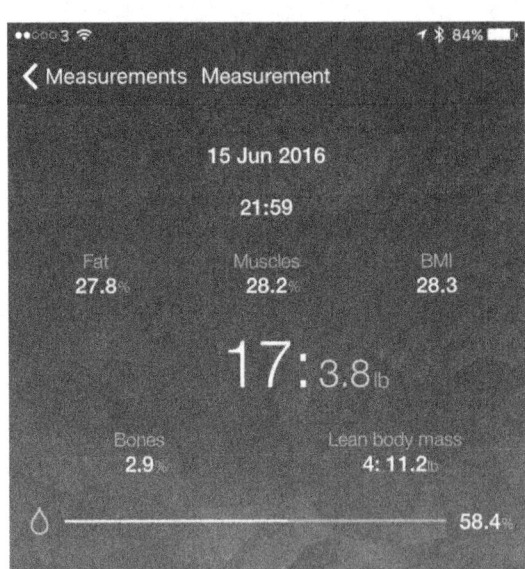

As you can see, I was a shade under 17st 4lb (110kg), was nearly 28% fat and my BMI was 28.3 which counts as overweight (and this was after losing a stone prior to buying the new scales).

Now here is my latest weigh-in:

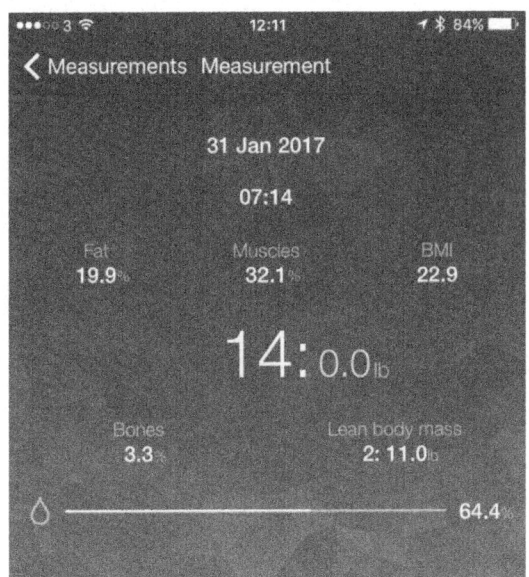

Figure 11 – My latest "Beets Blu" weigh in: 31 January 2017

I'm now 14st exactly (89kg), my body fat has dipped under 20% and my BMI at 22.9 is comfortably in the normal range. I've increased my muscle mass percentage, bone percentage and hydration levels.

My BMR

If you refer back to Figure 4 in Chapter Three you will see my initial BMR, which averaged out around 2,350ish. Here is my latest set of BMR data:

1,966	31 Jan 2017
2,061	30 Jan 2017
2,007	29 Jan 2017
2,085	28 Jan 2017
2,023	27 Jan 2017
1,979	26 Jan 2017
1,983	25 Jan 2017
2,018	24 Jan 2017
1,942	23 Jan 2017
2,058	22 Jan 2017
1,911	21 Jan 2017
1,966	20 Jan 2017
1,988	19 Jan 2017
1,915	18 Jan 2017

Figure 12 - My latest BMR data

You can see it has dropped down to around 2,000 or fewer calories per day, a 15% drop since I started.

My resting heart rate

So far so good. What about other health signs. Let's look at my heart rate (BPM) as recorded by my Apple Watch. Occasionally it returns an anomalous reading (as on 5 June and, to a lesser extent,

12 June in Figure 12). However, you can see that, on the whole, my watch is returning a minimum resting heart rate in the low 60bpm range.

Heart Rate	All Recorded Data	Edit
63 - 115		16 Jun 2016
61 - 140		15 Jun 2016
61 - 117		14 Jun 2016
63 - 104		13 Jun 2016
51 - 109		12 Jun 2016
65 - 107		11 Jun 2016
65 - 106		10 Jun 2016
68 - 112		9 Jun 2016
67 - 133		8 Jun 2016
60 - 98		7 Jun 2016
69 - 112		6 Jun 2016
41 - 110		5 Jun 2016
62 - 119		4 Jun 2016
61 - 99		3 Jun 2016

Figure 13 - My initial heart rate (BPM)

Now compare that to the last few days:

49 - 121	1 Feb 2017	
53 - 129	31 Jan 2017	
49 - 114	30 Jan 2017	
45 - 116	29 Jan 2017	
52 - 136	28 Jan 2017	
49 - 129	27 Jan 2017	
50 - 121	26 Jan 2017	
50 - 113	25 Jan 2017	
50 - 121	24 Jan 2017	
50 - 113	23 Jan 2017	
53 - 129	22 Jan 2017	
49 - 106	21 Jan 2017	
35 - 107	20 Jan 2017	
51 - 115	19 Jan 2017	

Figure 14 – My latest heart rate (BPM)

It's very clear (discounting a highly anomalous reading on 20 January) that my minimum resting heart rate has dropped by a good 10bpm.

What does this mean in practice?

A lower resting heart rate significantly reduces your risk of heart attack and stroke. This article in the Daily Telegraph explains more (http://www.telegraph.co.uk/science/2016/03/14/how-fast-your-heart-beats-predicts-if-you-will-die-early/). Most people's resting heart rate is between 60 and 100 bpm so as a result of this programme and regular exercise mine, at the age of 63 is in the low 50s and is closer to an athlete than an average person. I don't think I'm special and I haven't done any strenuous exercise or taken on any extreme eating fads.

It's just about creating a good routine and sticking to it (remember MAPS!!)

My blood pressure

Fortunately, I've always had reasonably low blood pressure and this hasn't changed much over the period of this programme. I have a decent home sphygmomanometer (I've always wanted to type that!) – blood pressure monitor to you and me – and here are the readings from last year:

109/64	29 Oct, 21:10
106/68	11 Oct, 21:21
105/57	22 Sep, 22:28
99/65	14 Sep, 21:21
107/65	10 Sep, 14:11
110/69	4 Sep, 20:59
95/58	28 Aug, 21:35
98/57	24 Aug, 21:56
97/60	14 Aug, 22:16
95/59	11 Aug, 20:05
112/72	3 Aug, 20:26
99/69	29 Jul, 19:43
99/65	27 Jul, 21:01
110/71	17 Jul, 08:52

Figure 15 – My blood pressure readings

As you can see, there has been very little change over the time period – 120/80 is considered normal; mine is verging on hypotensive (low blood pressure) but as I don't have any negative symptoms (dizziness etc.) it's nothing to worry about.

Measurements

When I started, my chest was 48 inches and my waist was 40 inches. They are now 42" and 34" respectively. I have had to renew my entire wardrobe (ouch!) but it has been so worthwhile. For the first time in years I have had the choice of mainstream fashion rather than just what's available in the outsize section. I can wear skinny jeans rather than baggy ones. I can go out with my shirt tucked in rather than over my stomach to hide it. And although I've had to replace all my clothes, I can actually choose from a much cheaper range rather than the expensive, hard to find stuff I used to have to buy.

So there you have it! I'm lighter, fitter, with a healthier heart and greater life expectancy – and after a year of relatively simple, straightforward and undemanding changes to my life. The important thing is to understand that this is a never ending journey. I have made some minor adjustments now I've reached my goal weight but nothing significant. I feel too good to want to change any of it anyway.

The last chapter in this book is simply a summary of everything that's gone before so we can bring all the elements together and allow you to use t as an *aide memoire* for when you need to refresh your memory or regain your moitivation.

Seven – Bringing it all together

Now you've read through the entire programme, let's summarise all the different elements in one place, just so you get the full picture.

I think of this a bit like a jigsaw puzzle – you need all the pieces but you also need the picture on the box to know where to put them!

The different elements

Here are the different elements:

1. Know what your "core" weight is – it isn't a fixed data point it's a range
    a. A good set of scales will help and, if you can afford it, get a set of Wi-Fi or Bluetooth scales that will record all your data for you
2. Know your BMR (and remember that it reduces as you lose weight)
3. Weigh daily – accept the fluctuations and learn your body rhythms

4. Know your Basal Metabolic Rate (BMR)
    a. You can find online calculators to help you
    b. Don't forget it reduces as you lose weight – recheck regularly alongside your weight loss
5. Commit to a daily active calorie goal – and stick to it
    a. Again, don't forget that, as you lose weight, your calorie burn will decrease with the same level of exercise. You will need to accept that your weight loss will slow down or you will need to increase your exercise target or reduce your calorie intake if you want to maintain the same level of weight loss
6. Create a diet that works for you – are you a morning or evening eater. What proteins do you like (as they digest more slowly and keep you full longer. Learn to ask yourself the question "Is it worth the calories?" For me, wine was "yes" but chocolate was "no". It will almost certainly be different for you.
7. Have a "go-to" food when you really need to eat but don't want to wreck your day's efforts. For me it was a Pink Lady apple but it could be a bowl of vegetable soup or a cereal bar. Keep asking "Is it worth the calories?"
8. Have an exercise plan and stick to it. If you can't walk to work, can you get off the bus or the train one stop or two stops earlier and walk the rest. Can you park the car a bit

further away? Anything that encourages you to walk a bit further each day is a marginal gain!

9. Plan to do a bit more at the weekends. Discover your local community. Go to places you haven't been to. Broaden your mind!
10. Track your data. Whether it's a Fitbit, Apple watch or an online resource, the ability to look back and compare is priceless. Look at all the examples in this book. It continually motivates me to keep on track when I see the progress I have made. It will work for you too.

So there we have it. MY simple, straightforward "this is not a diet" book.

In ending, I just want to say a little bit more about the effect this programme has had on me, my wife and our relationship.

Between us we have now lost seven and a half stone (the weight of a human being). We are healthier, more active, go out more, do more things together, have a better relationship, laugh more, eat healthier and spend less on our food (very few take-aways). Food tastes better.

I really hope you get the same benefits as we did. I am positive that, if you follow the simple advice in this book, and you really want to make this change, you will be successful. In fact it is impossible not to be if you do follow these steps. They HAVE to work. The numbers prove it!

Printed in Dunstable, United Kingdom